THE PICTURE BOOK OF

MOTHERS

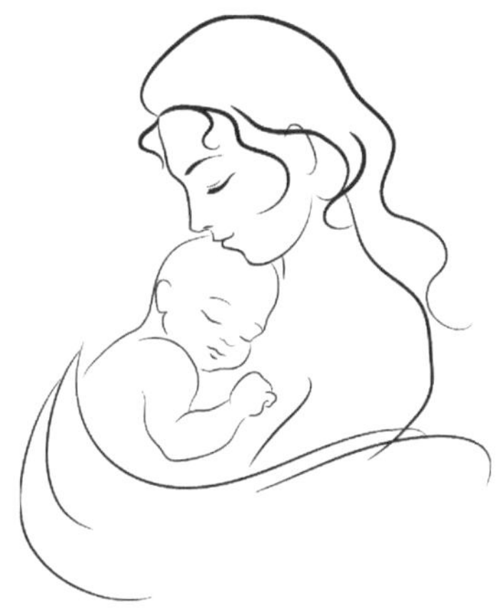

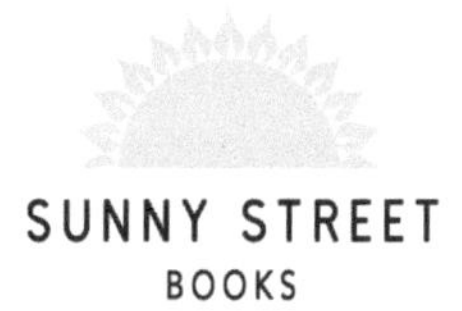

SUNNY STREET
BOOKS

Of all the gifts life has to offer, a loving mother is the greatest of them all.

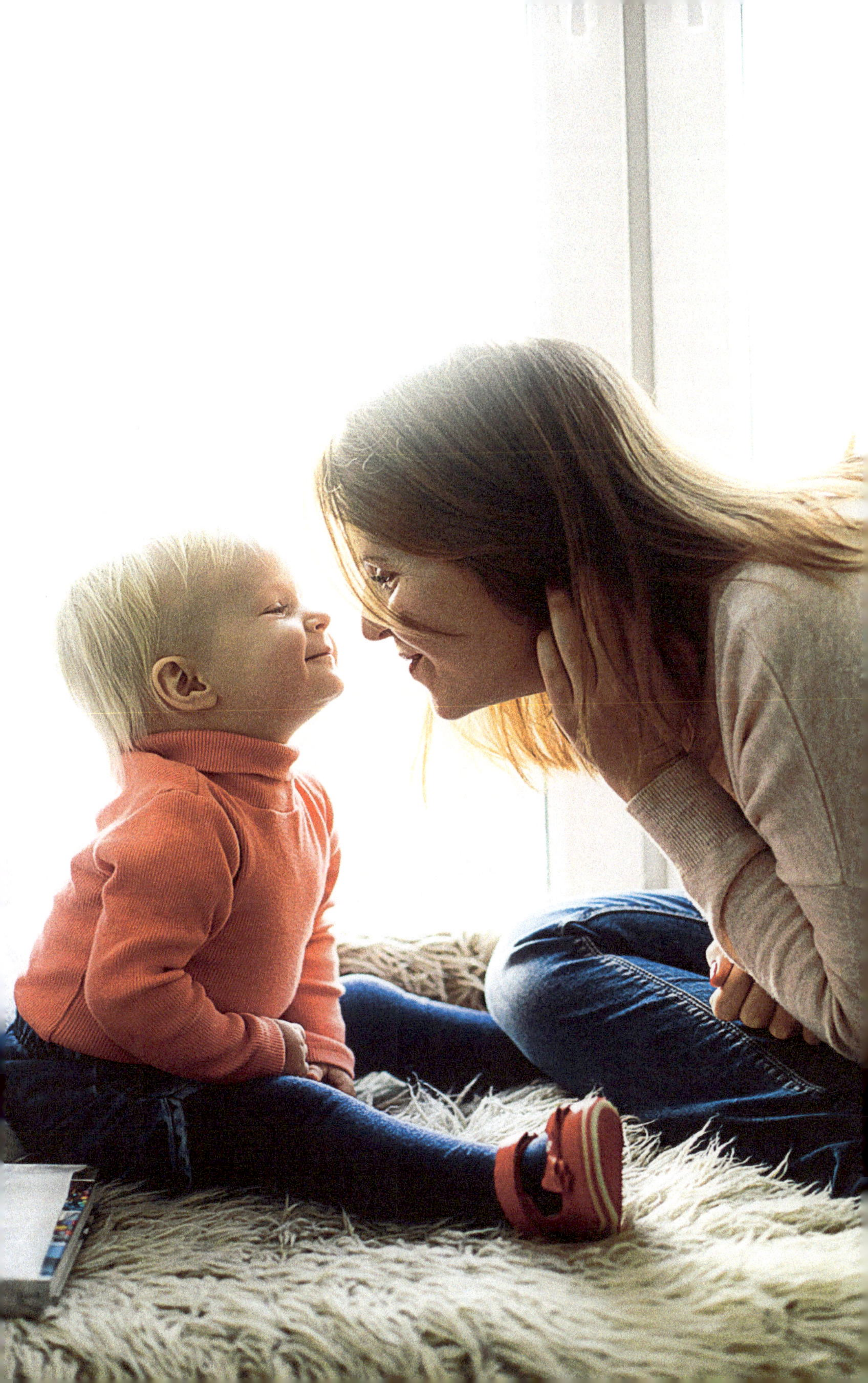

Mother and child never truly part. Maybe in distance, but never in heart.

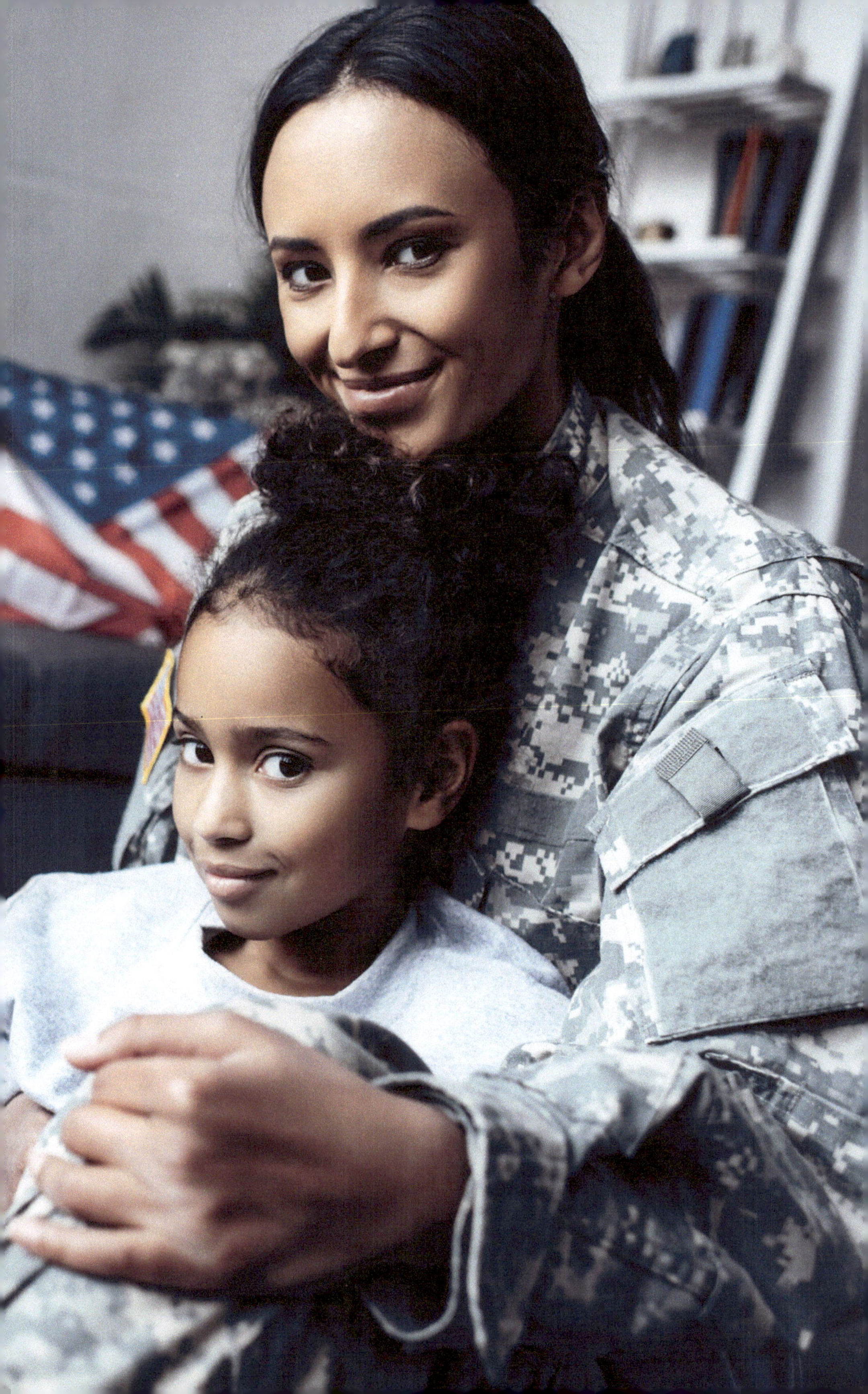

Life doesn't come with an instruction manual. It comes with a mother.

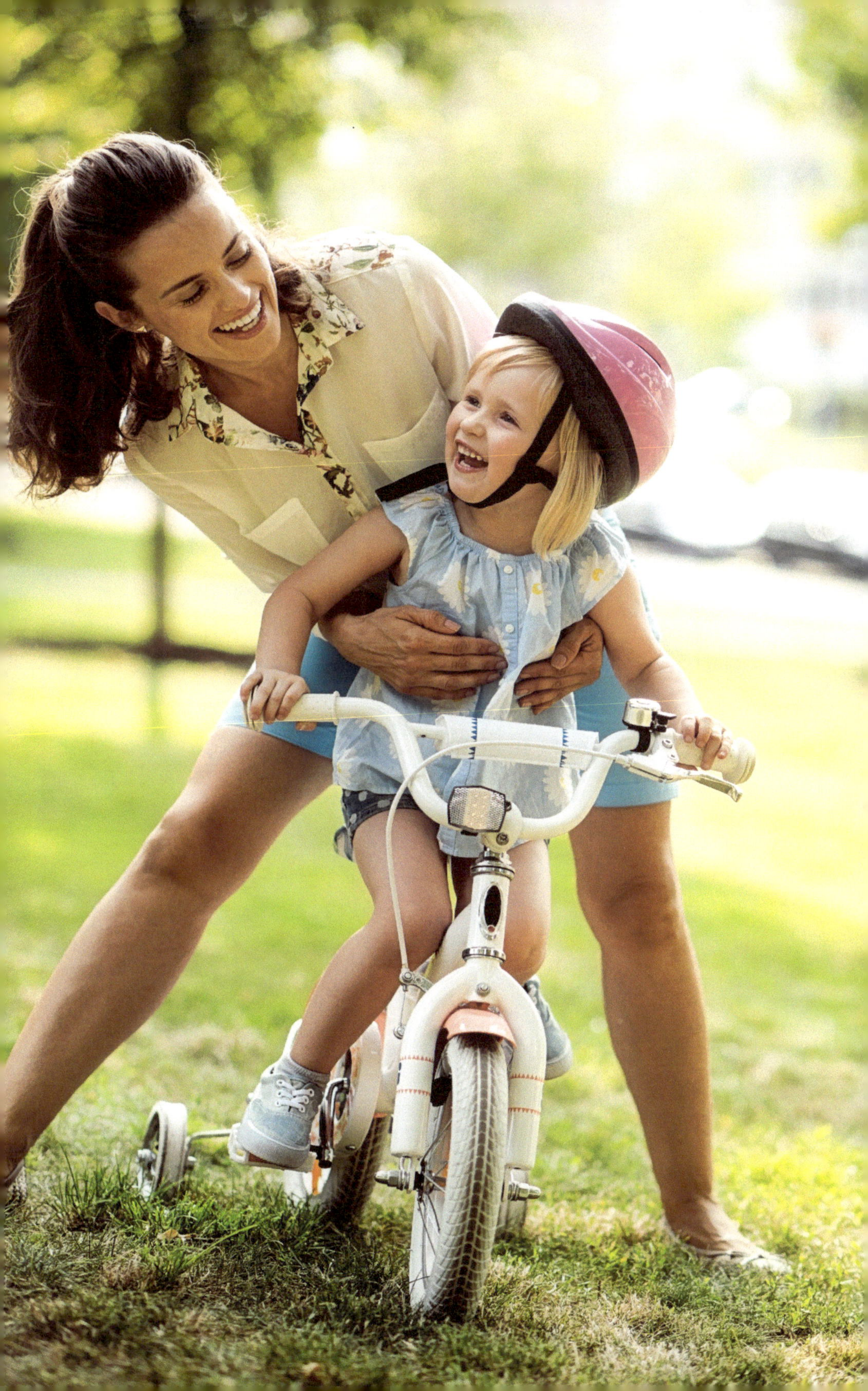

A mother is your first friend, your best friend, your forever friend.

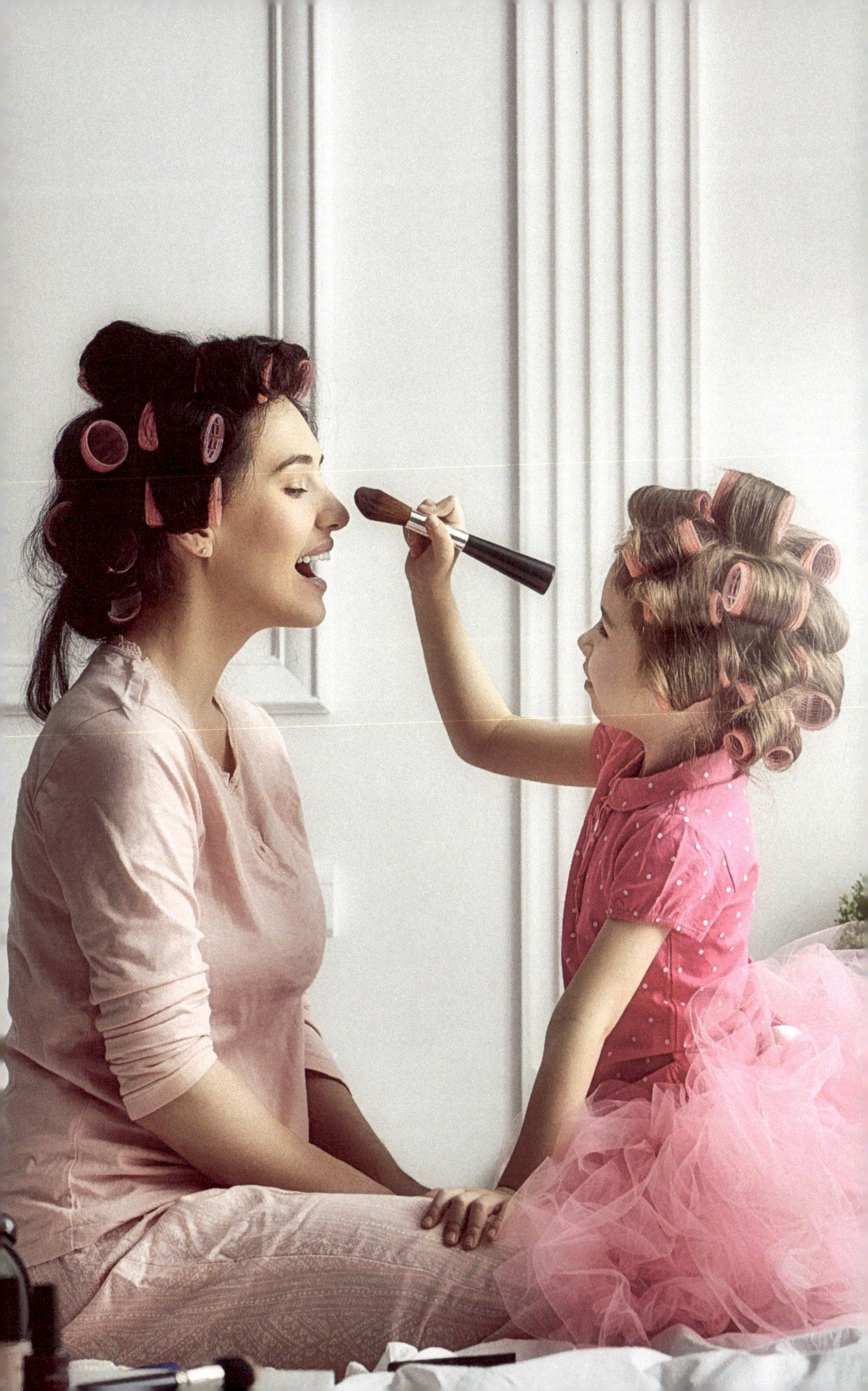

A mother's arms

are more comforting

than anyone else's.

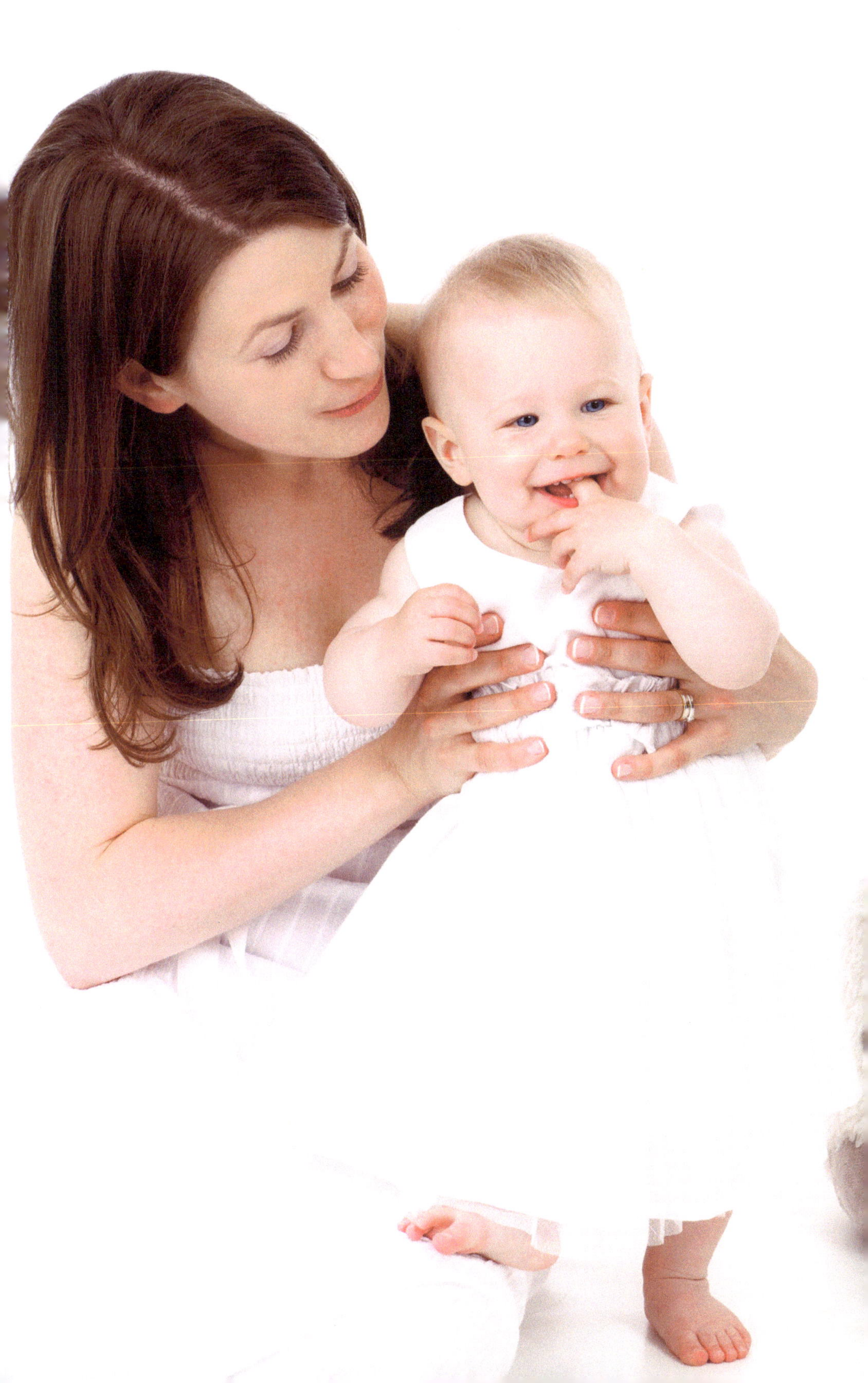

A mom's hug

lasts long after she

lets go.

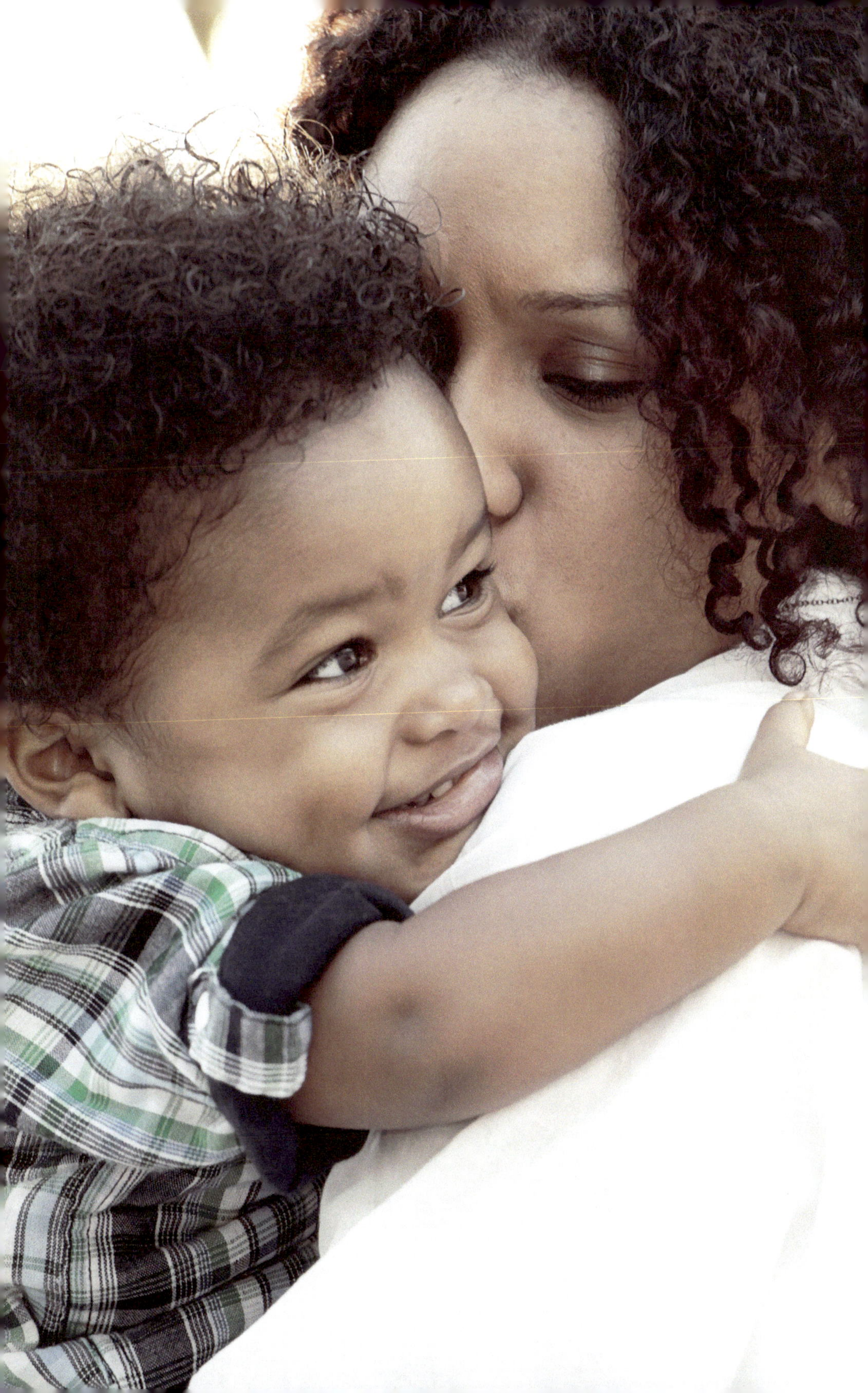

A mother is
someone you laugh
with, dream with,
and love with all
your heart.

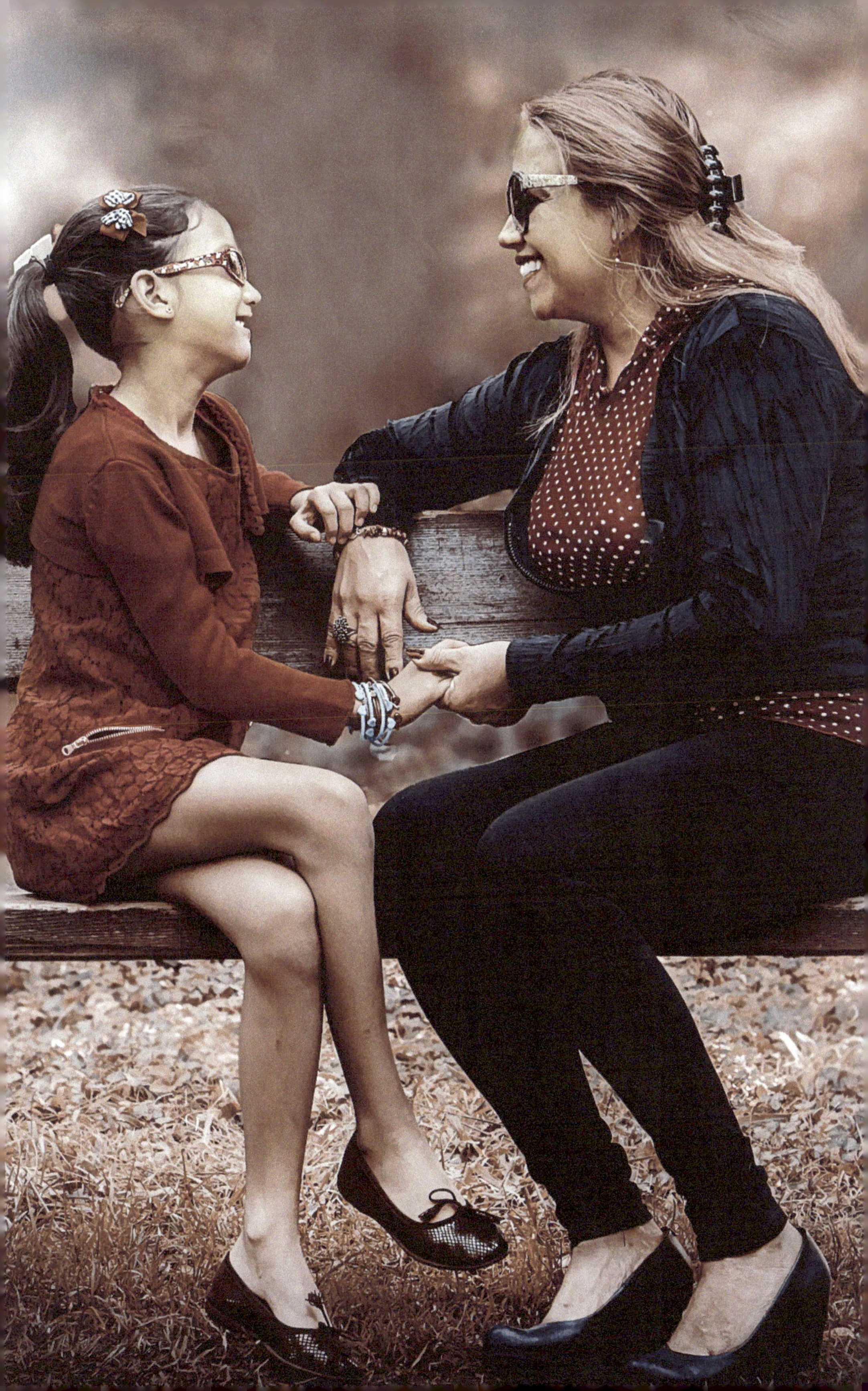

The love between

a mother and child

lasts forever.

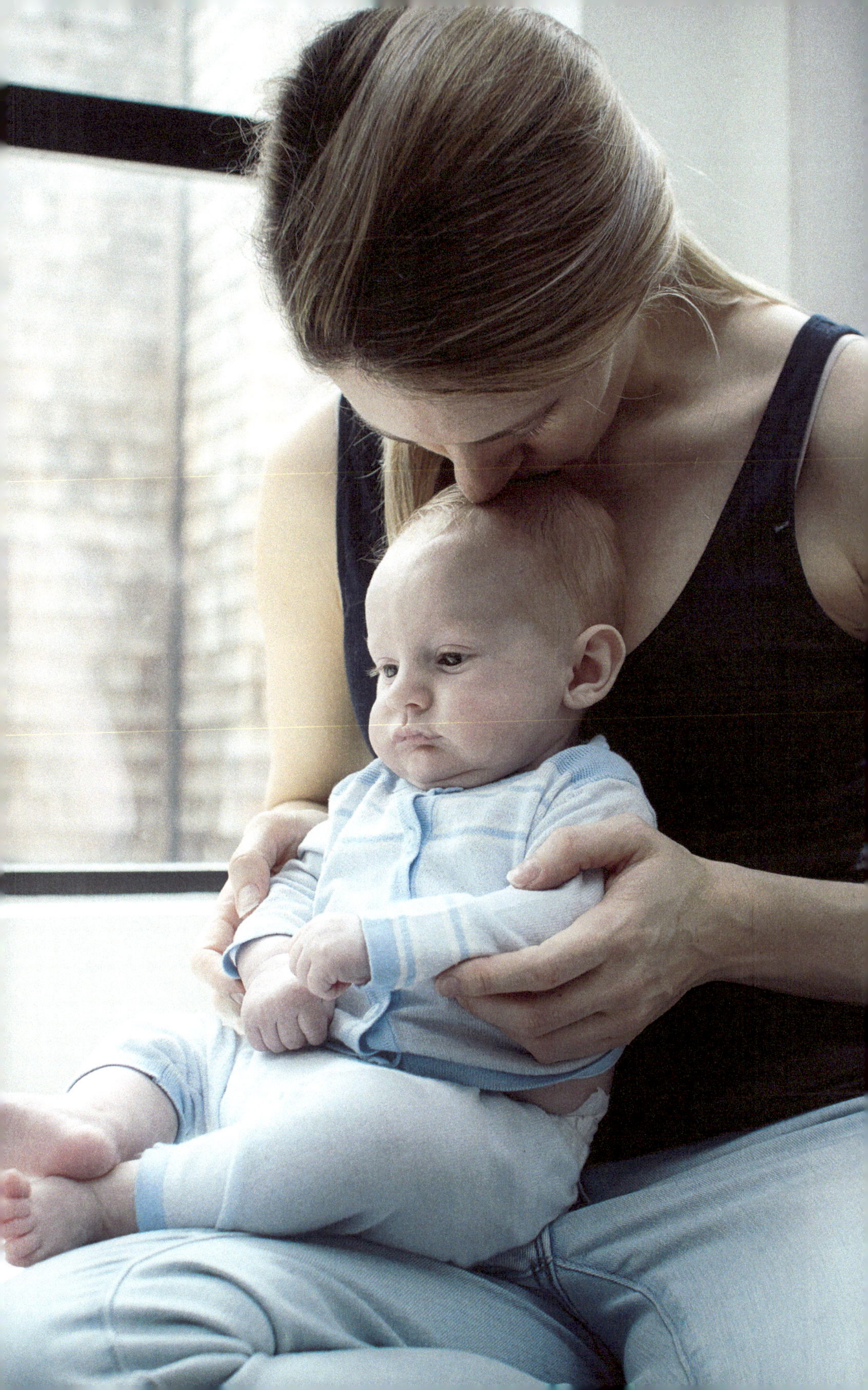

God could not be
everywhere, so he
made mothers.

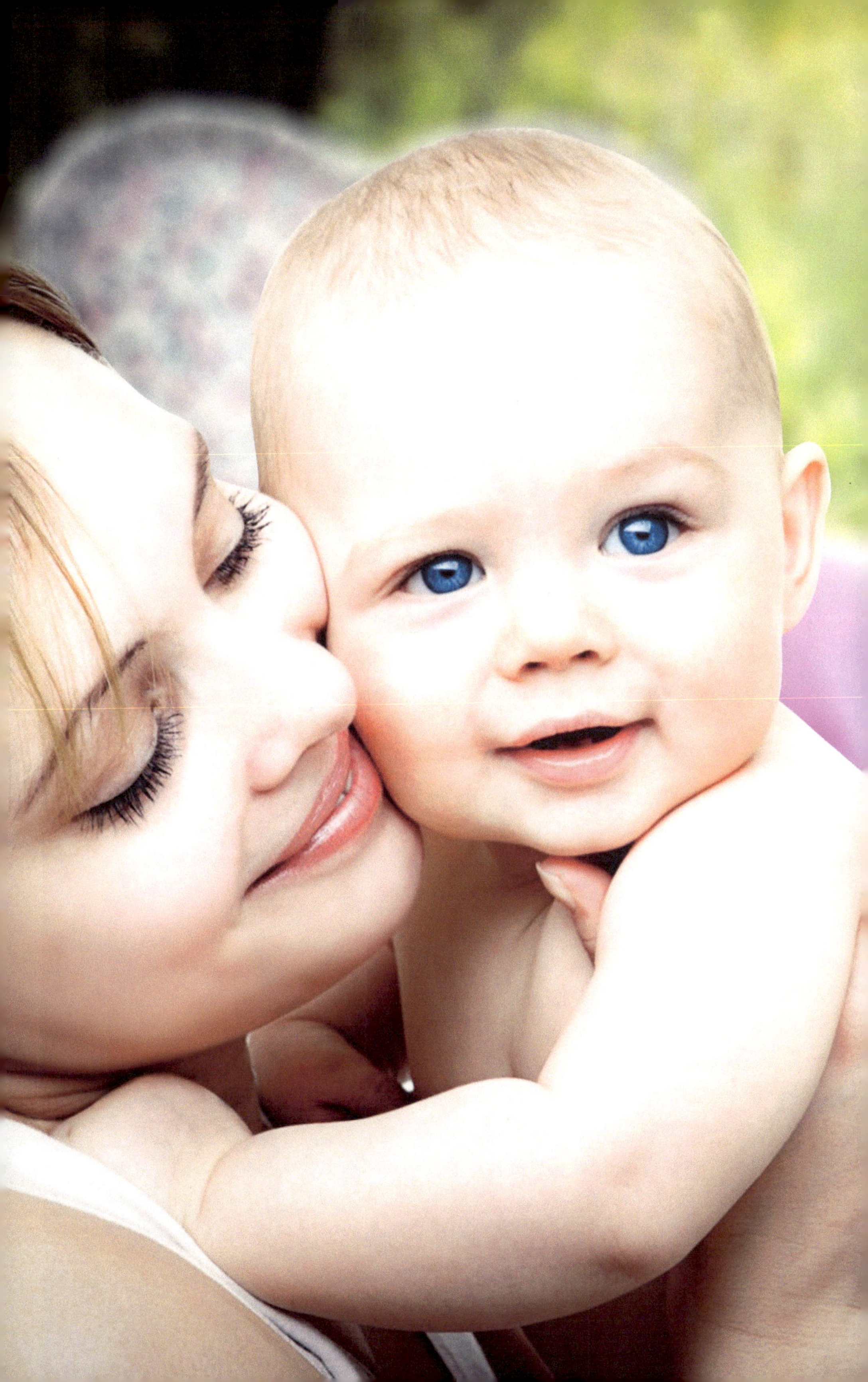

Mothers never run out of hugs and cookies.

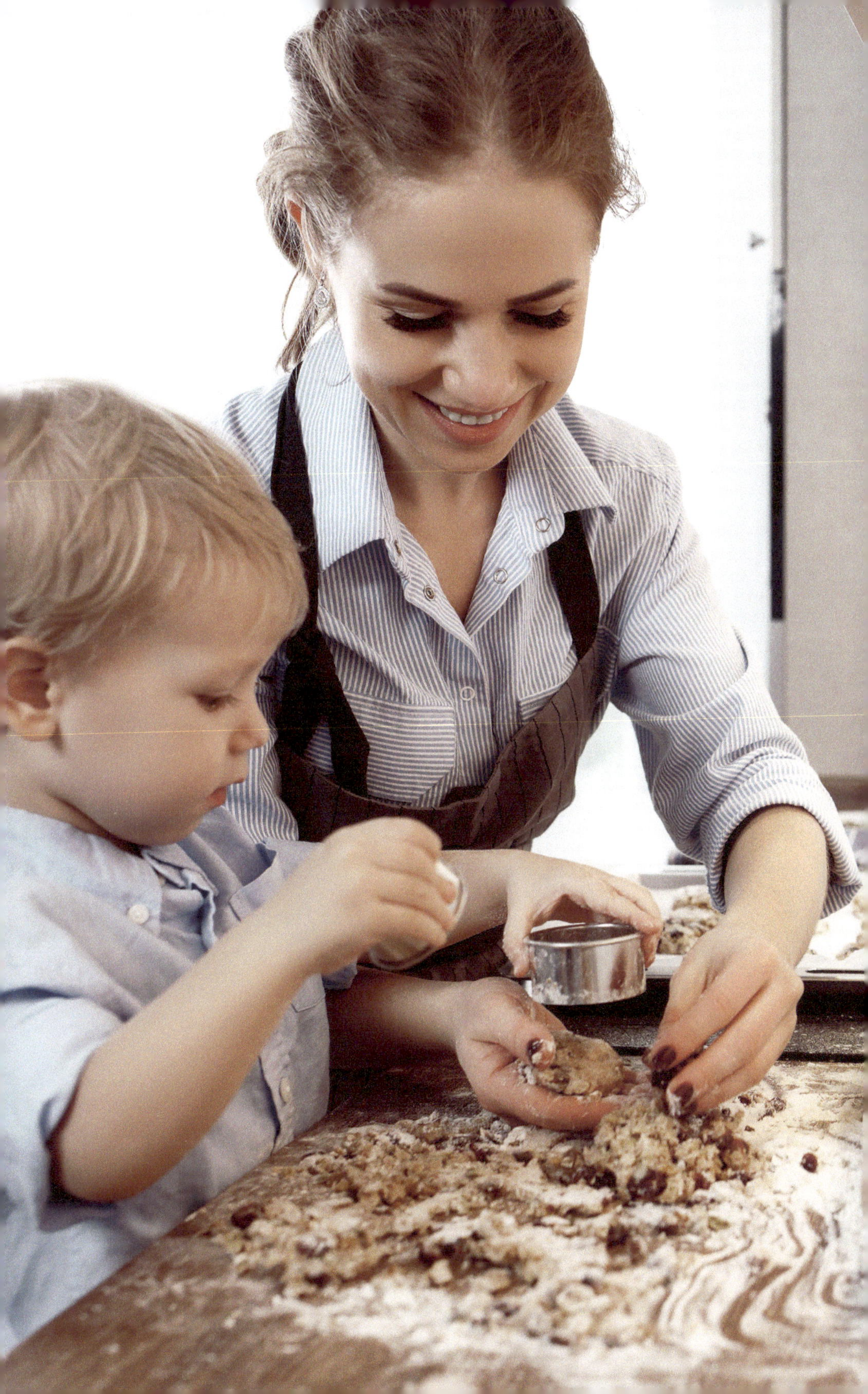

A child

outgrows a mother's

lap but never her

heart.

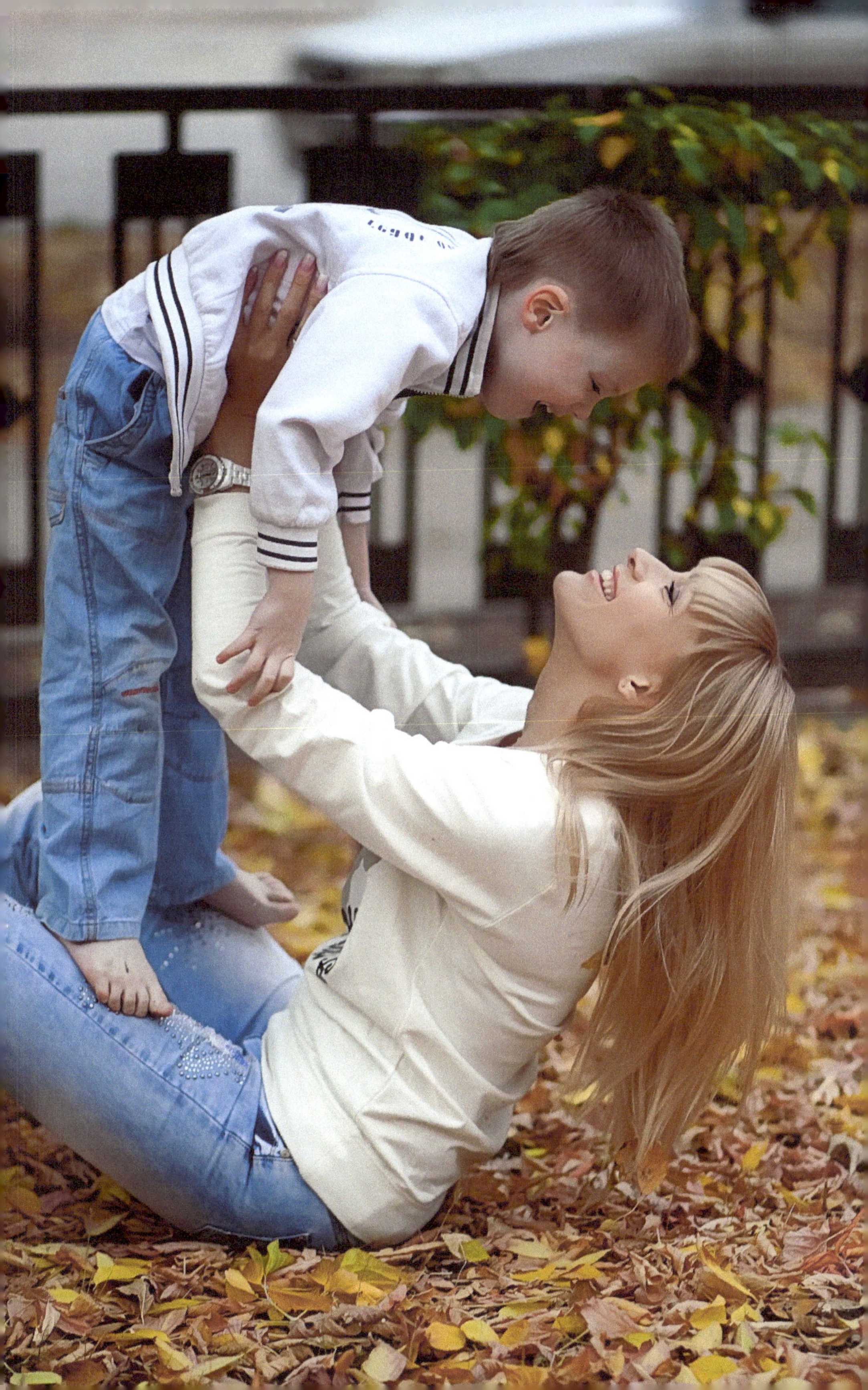

$\mathcal{A}$ man's work is
from sun to sun, but
a mother's work is
never done.

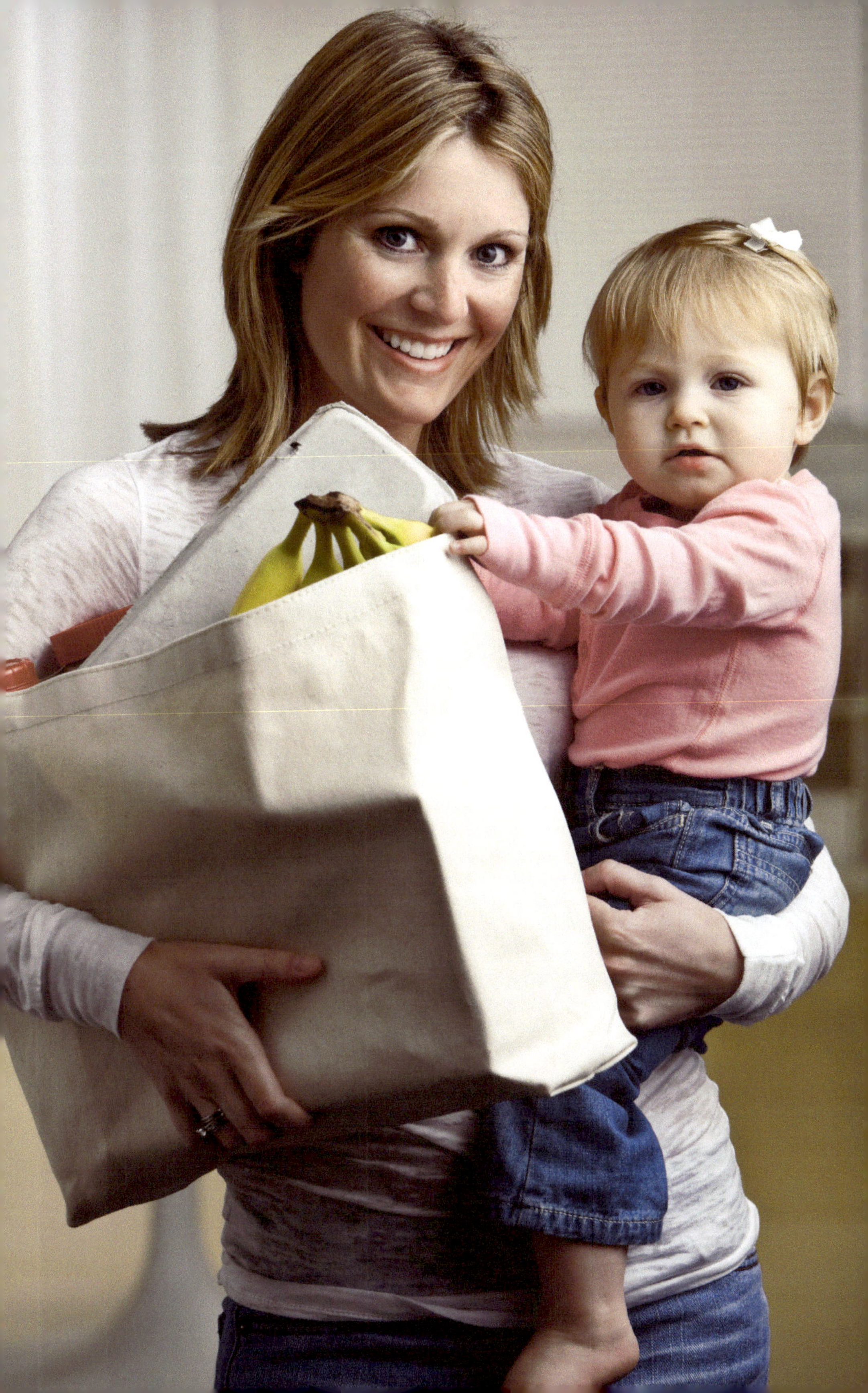

The highest and
noblest work in this
life is that of a
mother.

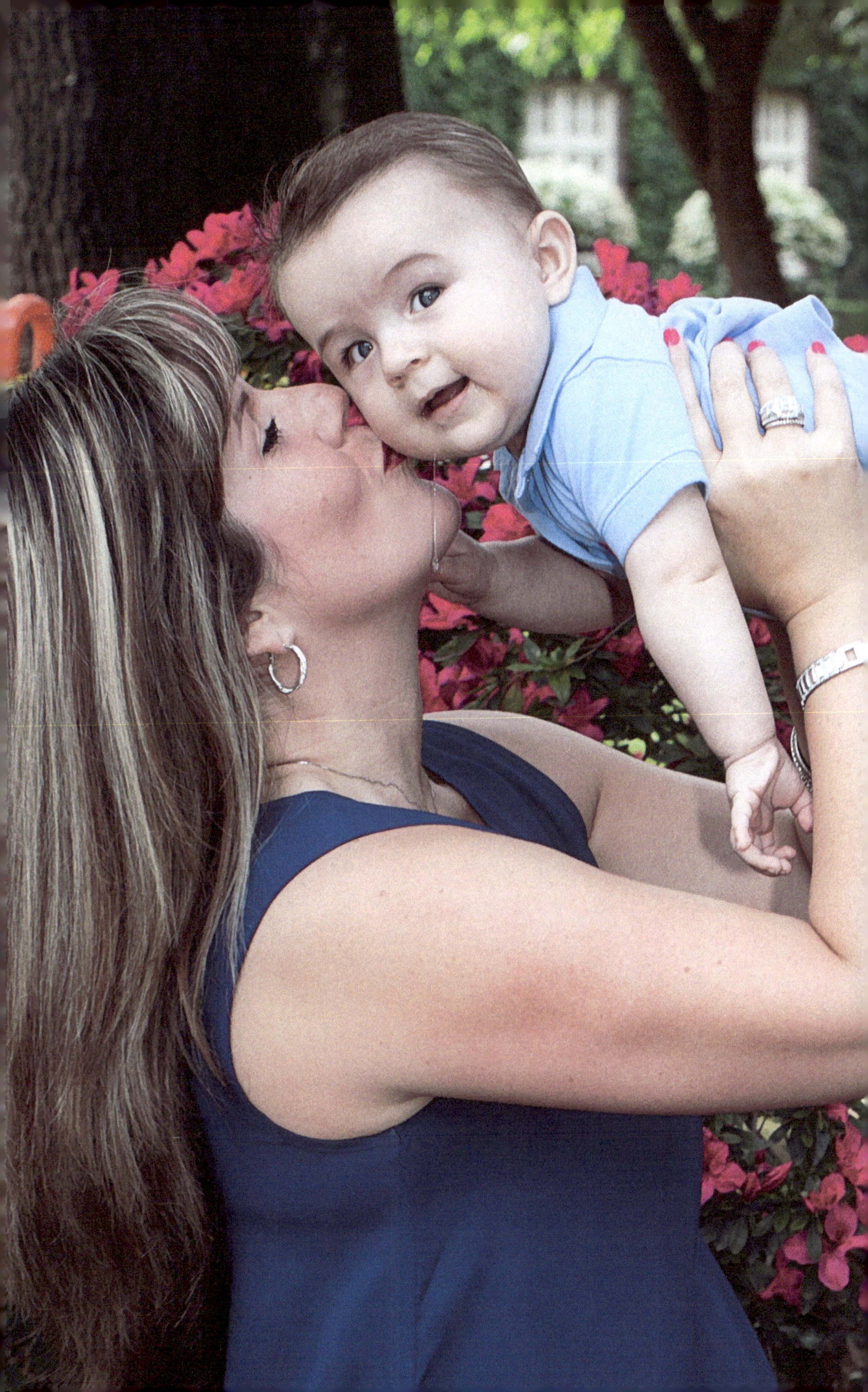

$\mathcal{T}$o the world you
are a mother, but to
your child you are
the world.

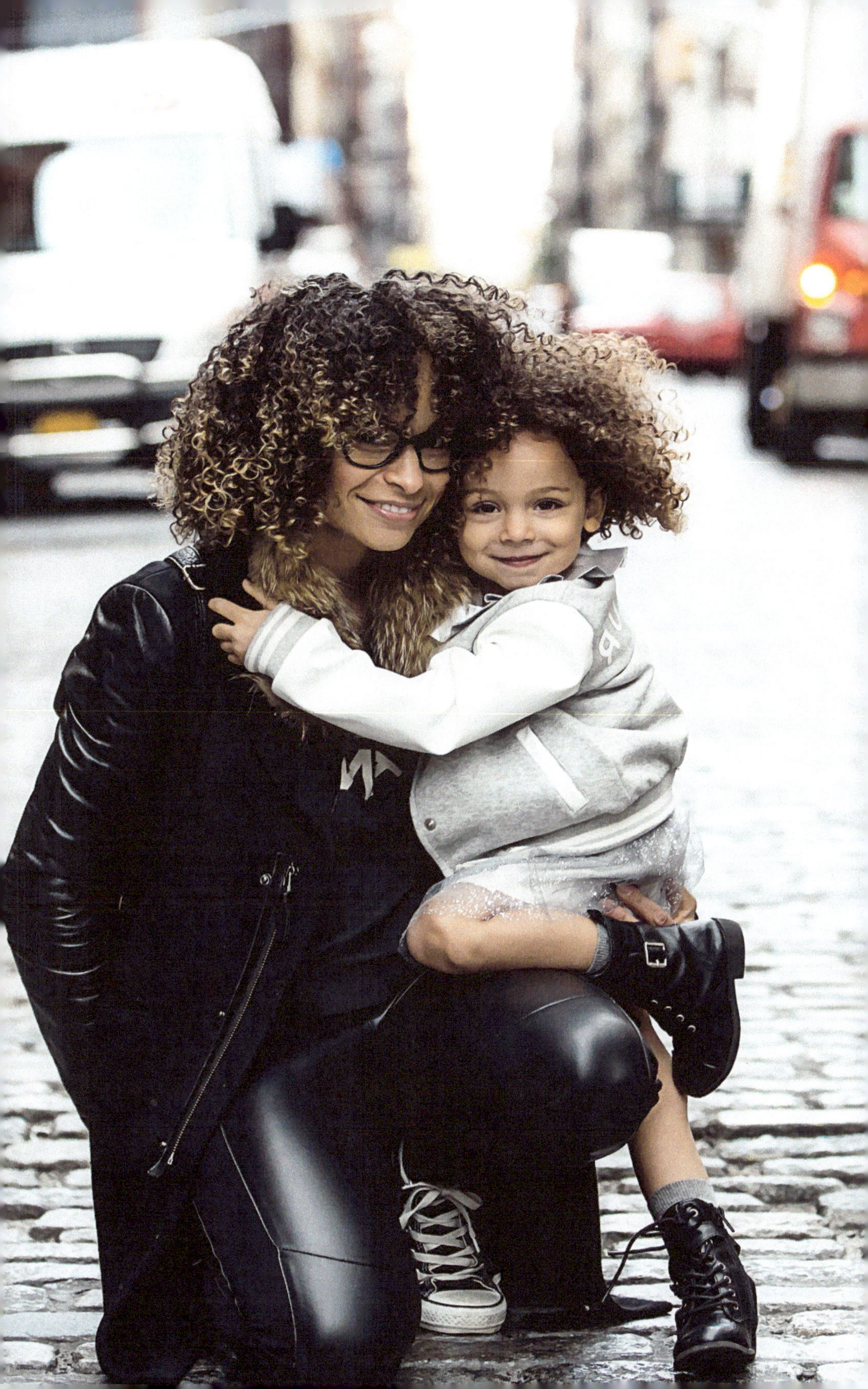

There's no way to

be a perfect mother,

but a million ways

to be a good one.

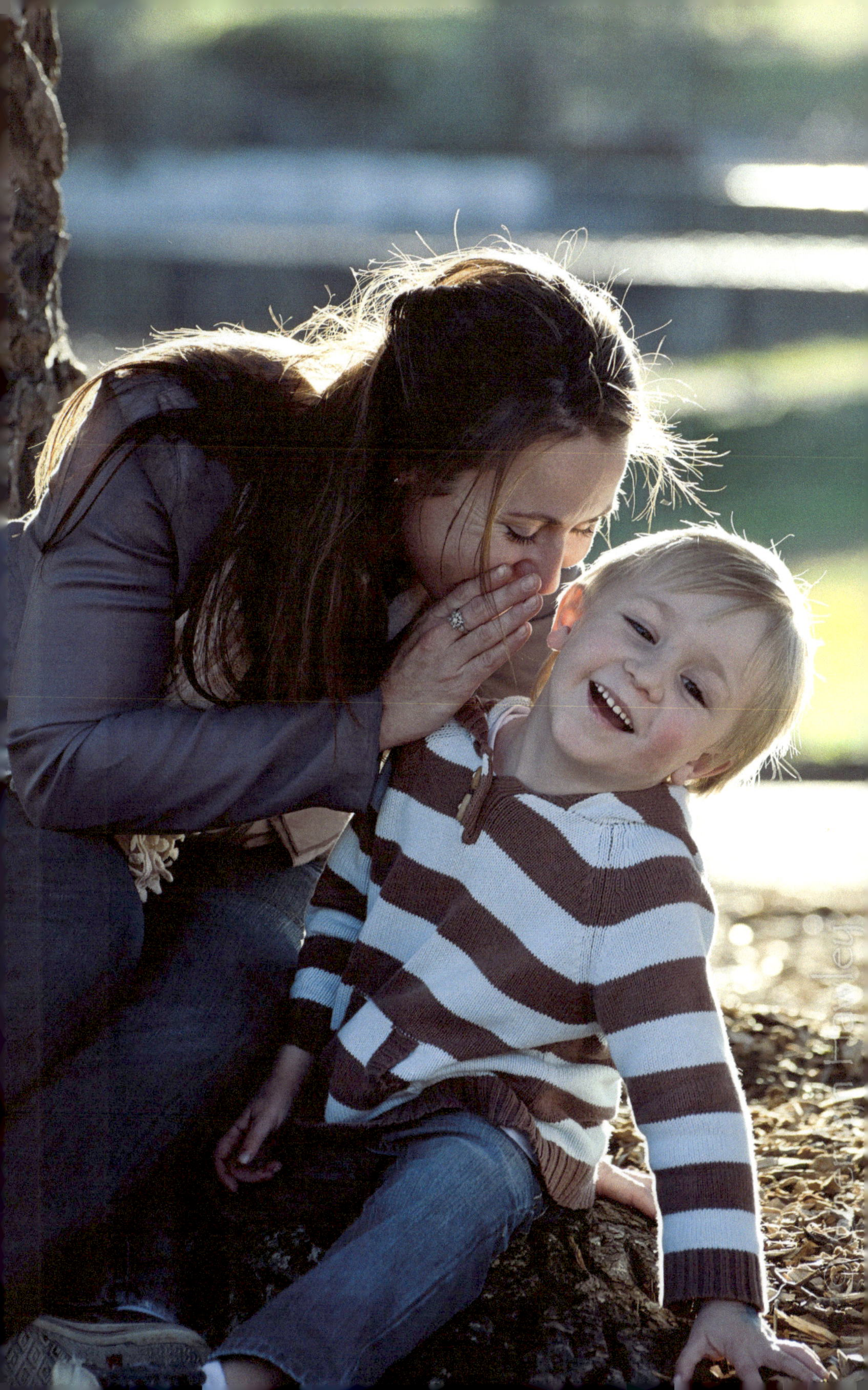

A mother's hug

lasts long after she

lets go.

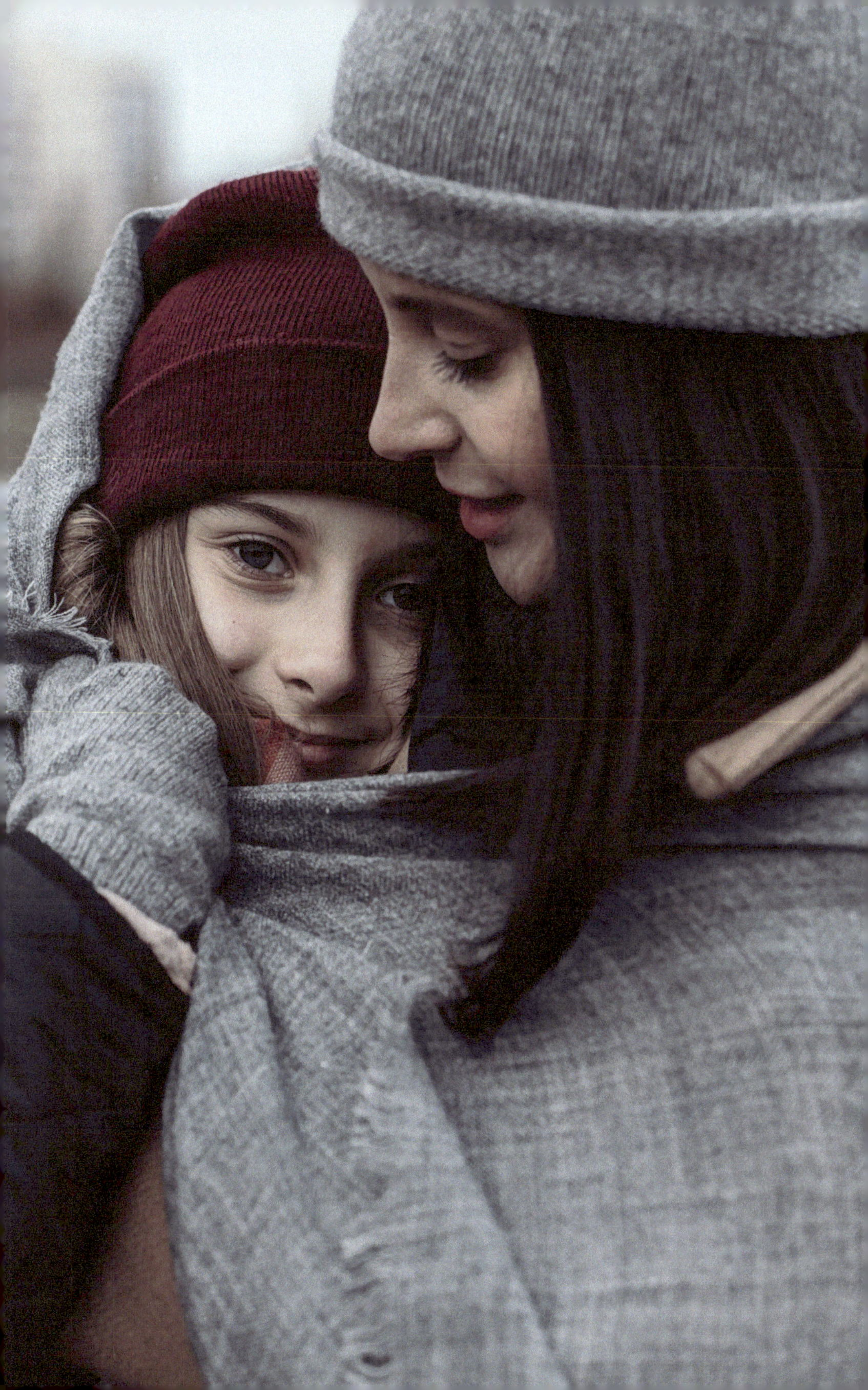

$\mathcal{A}$ mother is she
who can take the
place of all others
but whose place no
one else can take.

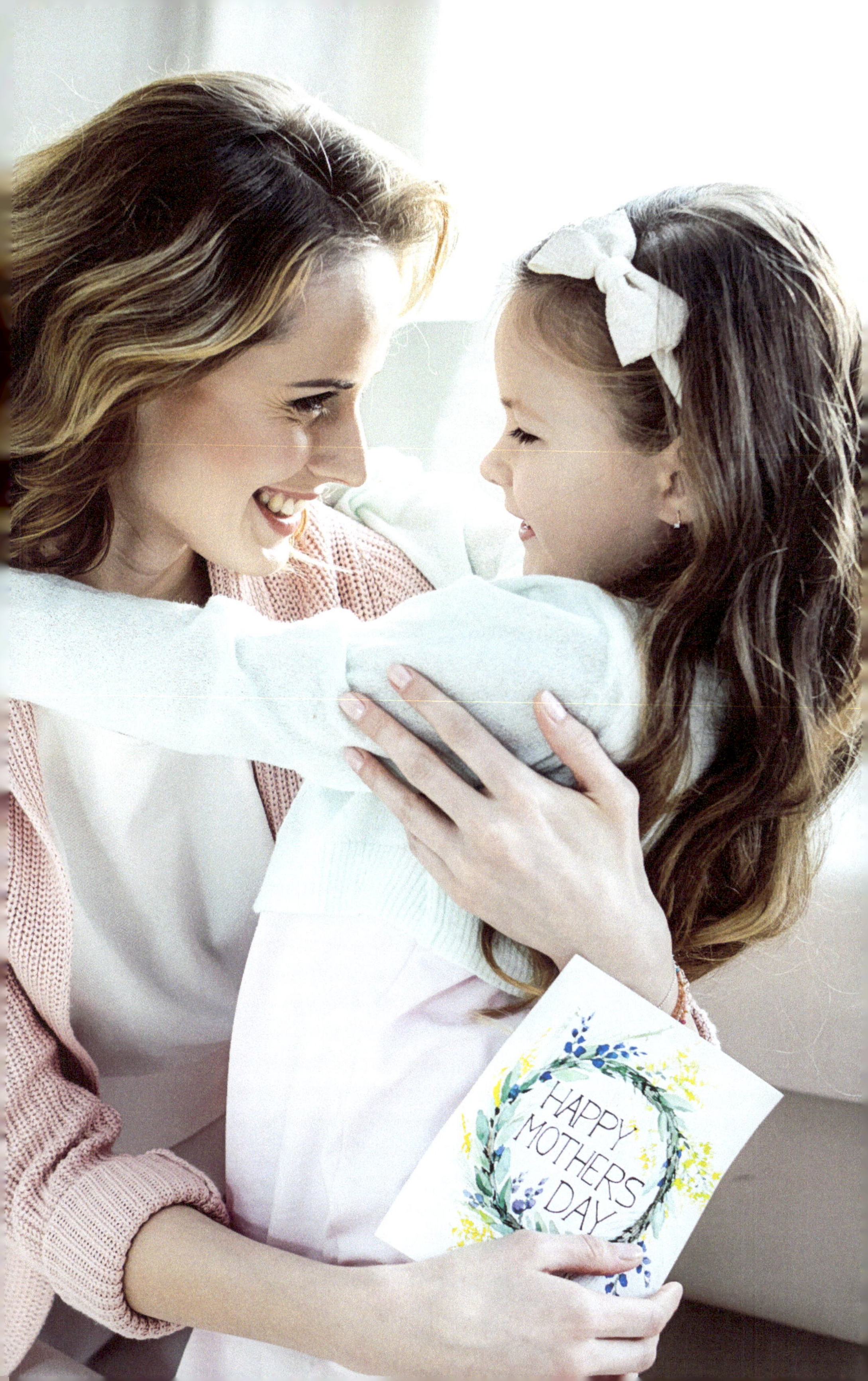
HAPPY
MOTHERS
DAY

$\mathcal{M}$oms are like buttons. They hold everything together.

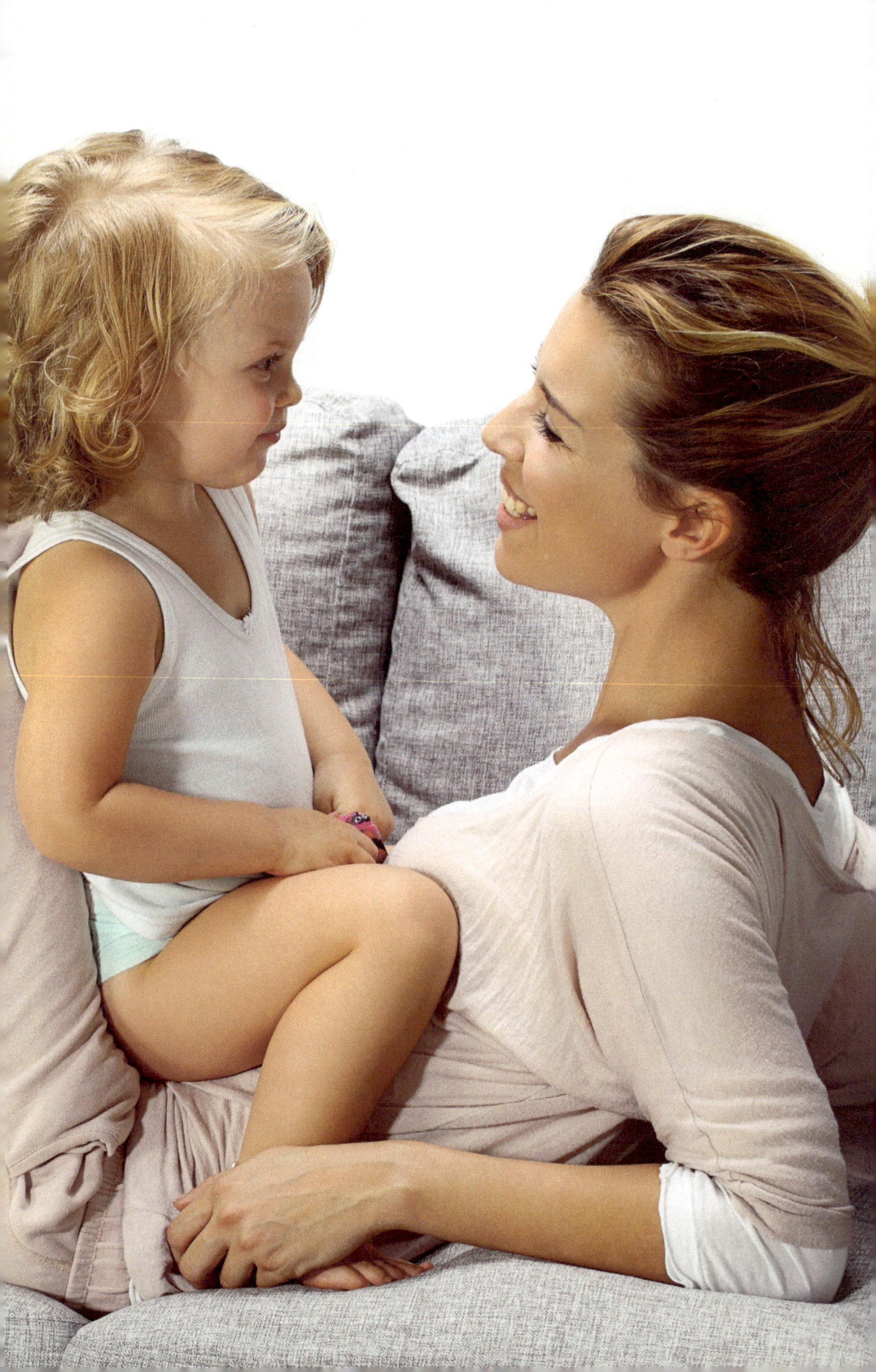

$\mathcal{M}$others never
sleep. They just
worry with their
eyes open.

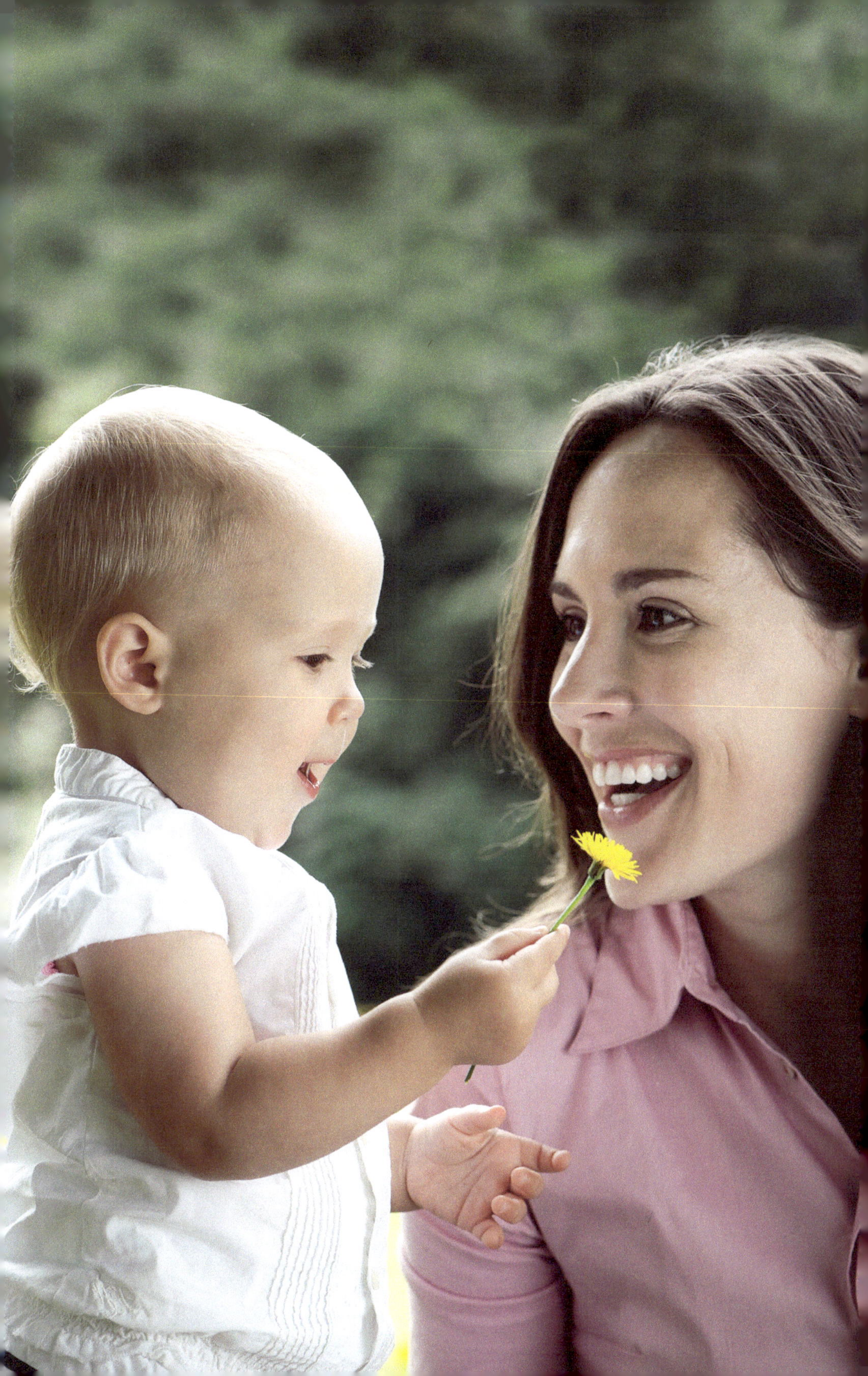

*M*otherhood:

All love begins and

ends there.

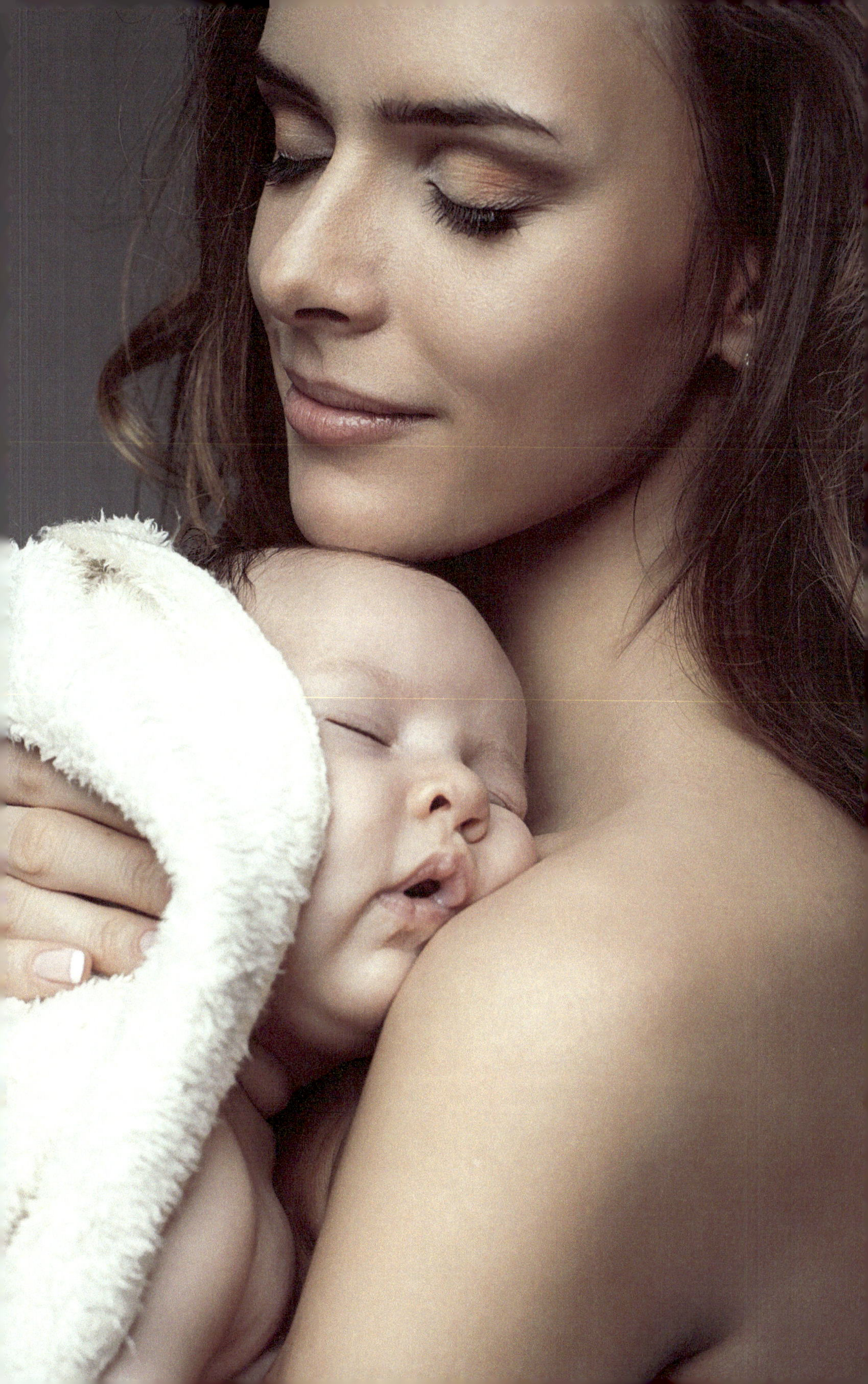